MW01227317

21 Days of Eating Mindfully

Your Guide to a Healthy Relationship with Yourself and Food

BY LORRIE JONES, MBSR BSN CYI

Every effort has been made to ensure that the information contained in this book is complete and accurate. However, neither the publisher nor the author is engaged in rendering professional advice or services to the individual reader. The ideas and suggestions in this book are not intended as a substitute for consulting with your physician. All matters regarding health require medical supervision. Neither the author nor the publisher shall be liable or responsible for any loss, injury or damage allegedly arising from any information or suggestion in this book.

Content by Lorrie Jones, Founder, Simple Serenity LLC

Logo design by Nikki Cole, nikkicolecreative.com

Editorial and book layout by Kelly Lenihan, ksldesigns.com

SECOND EDITION: PUBLISHED IN THE UNITED STATES OF AMERICA

ISBN-13: 978-1468112092

ISBN-10: 1468112090

About the Author

LORRIE JONES, MBSR BSN CYI

Mindfulness based programs and practices are my signature work, my professional joy. As the only person in Washington State certified to teach Mindfulness Based Stress Reduction (MBSR), I offer a conscious, creative and compassionate approach to personal renewal and mindful practices for health and well-being. As a wellness practitioner, educator and coach, I have served individuals, groups, and hospitals with my expertise in health issues, with a specialty in the area of eating behaviors. In my work, I help people believe their life is worth being present for, building the strength it takes to no longer consider doing anything less than what is in their very best interest.

Following two decades of research and practical experience, I developed a 21-day program, *21 Days of Eating Mindfully,* designed to encourage and support women in changing unwanted and unhealthy eating habits by transforming their relationship with themselves.

This 21 day journey is not a diet or an overnight cure. Rather, it is an opportunity to inquire more deeply within, providing the keys to establishing a healthy, loving relationship with yourself and enjoying a favorable weight shift and wise eating choices as a natural result and a sustainable outcome. With mindful awareness, it is possible to let go of the belief that eating or not eating will take away hurt, disappointment, loneliness – boredom, anger, emptiness. With mindful awareness, you will stop using food for anything other than nourishment and healthy enjoyment.

CR

HERE'S WHAT PEOPLE ARE SAYING

"This 21-day process is SO thorough; I like the quotes inserted throughout. Journaling can be very powerful; it helps me be aware of daily events connected with food: I don't eat enough during the day and by dinnertime, I'm starved. Following daily prompts is non-threatening – like having a friend that I'm talking to. 21 days is doable and supports people to take time for themselves and become aware of everything they put in their mouth."

—M. B., Spokane, WA

"Having edited this book, I'm quite familiar with the content. However, after following the 21-day guide from the reader's perspective, I am astonished at how much I learned about myself. Powerful information to be armed with, for sure! I can now take this information and make better choices, redirect my emotional responses in healthier ways and simply be more mindful in the kitchen. This book provides valuable insights and tools and I highly recommend it to anyone struggling with their relationship with food, weight or self-image. Mindfulness and self-awareness goes beyond how one eats, it's a life style, and this book holds the key to a healthier you."

—K. L., Kirkland, WA

"Learning to let go of food numbing my feelings, my thoughts and my life was challenging – but it was possible. This 21-day journey exemplifies Lorrie's expertise, compassion and caring. She knows her work and brings her heart to everything she does."

—A. N., Woodinville, WA

"This is a beautiful, compassionate and extremely helpful book. Although it's written for women, I think so much of it can be used by men as well. Lorrie leads the reader through a series of gentle and easy to follow day-by-day steps. Firstly, she explores the day's topic, such as Hunger & Healing, Empathy & Emotional Eating, Awareness & Acceptance, Love & Letting Be, Inquiry & Intention, Nurture & Nourishment, and Gratitude & Gracious Living. Next, she offers a Mindfulness Activity, which includes many thoughtful and investigative questions regarding one's beliefs about food, body, self-worth and the stories we tell ourselves, to name a few. Then, she encourages the reader to take a bit of time and write down responses to the day's Mindfulness Activity, often providing wonderfully evocative questions to spur one's writing along such as " Am I hungry for nourishment or for something deeper?" Or, "What challenges can you name that contain the gift of joy?" The videos and handouts provide additional support and resources on the path to becoming more aware in the present moment around issues with food and body. I love this book. More than ever before, I'm able to recognize feelings as they emerge, stay with that awareness and allow myself to make different choices. This, to me, is freedom. I highly recommend this to anyone who wants to change their relationship to food, but more importantly, I highly recommend this book to those who want to change their relationship to themselves."

—A. F., Seattle, WA

CR

Table of Contents

ᘒ

Dedication

> *"When I write about hunger, I am really writing about love and the hunger for it, and warmth and the love of it and the hunger for it...and then the warmth and richness and fine reality of hunger satisfied...and it is all one."*
>
> —M.F.K. Fisher

My life is a journey which has led me here, to you. I've gained and lost over 1,900 pounds in my lifetime. By learning to eat mindfully and intuitively, I have not only healed my own relationship with food, I have changed my entire life. This book is dedicated to my family, my children and grandchildren, my teachers, my clients and to my dear friend and creative genius, Kelly Lenihan. Because of the support and lessons learned from each of you, I am able to share this rich program with women everywhere. *21 Days of Eating Mindfully* is dedicated to every woman who has ever struggled with her weight, her relationship with herself and with food.

In my own journey, I have discovered that my passion is helping others do the same. If you are at the beginning of your journey toward health and well-being and are looking for support, please visit www.simpleserenity.com for information on individual and group programs and helpful resources.

Healthy living starts today! *Are you ready?*

CS

Introduction: 21 Days of Eating Mindfully

> *"You are that which you seek."*
>
> — St. Francis

If you are like most women, you spend your days juggling many roles, conflicting commitments and the wants and needs of others. Often you come last, if there's time. The temptation to reach for food can be overwhelming. Eating emotionally can become a way of life and compulsive behavior can become an attempt to manage feelings only to have the compulsions manage us in the end.

When a pattern of compulsive overeating, emotional eating, under-eating or rigid dieting or control is established, we often believe the "problem" is about the struggle: the endless loyalty and dedication we create pushing ourselves to be better, thinner, different from who we are. While we may have succeeded in changing certain behaviors — perhaps even losing some weight — we have failed to understand and experience the deep level of change necessary for healing, growth and lifetime health.

The true cause of our months, years and perhaps a lifetime of struggle with weight is that we have forgotten who we truly are and have, instead, allowed fear, shame and guilt to run our lives. We have forgotten how to trust ourselves, how to trust our lives and how to live joyfully. We have forgotten the power of paying attention mindfully and in doing so, we turn to our compulsions — to food or to control — to numb ourselves rather than experience fully what we are feeling.

CR

Our true hunger is for something beneath the tyranny of diets and control. We are hungry for a deeply authentic life — a life lived with purpose, joy, passion and freedom. We are starving for a deep and abiding relationship with our true selves — one that brings us alive and one that is loving, compassionate and forgiving.

It has been reported that 95 to 98 percent of all the weight lost in the United States is gained back in a year to a year and a half — often with even more weight added on than before. Diets don't work because they are based on inadequacy and brokenness. Diets imply there is something wrong with us and that we need fixing. Fear and inadequacy are not respectable motivators and willpower and deprivation are not sustainable behavioral plans. Rather, healing must come from a deeper level than the problem of excess weight or undesirable eating habits. Healing must involve not only the body but the mind, emotions and spirit. And when there is deep healing, all of life is in a natural balance — including weight. When we open to what has been closed, look directly at what has been hidden, and remember what we have forgotten, we begin to see our unwanted eating habits as guides and our worries and obstacles as gifts — a doorway into the healing that we long for and dream of.

Welcome to this guide, designed to offer you 21 days of inquiry, inspiration and encouragement in healing from unhealthy eating habits. Each day will begin with a few words, some points to ponder and suggestions for simple, mindful activities to focus awareness and attention. Action and involvement are imperative because eating compulsions cannot be solved on a mental level only. Please feel free to use the pages in any way you wish,

CR

bypassing questions if you desire and/or re-asking others. Your responses may change moment to moment! I encourage you to record your thoughts in a personal journal so that you can look back on your notes as a resource.

The intention of this guidebook is not to offer advice or attempt to make you "better". Rather, this book is an introduction meant to inspire and guide you as you delve into the mindfulness activities and journal prompts. I encourage you to let each day's inquiries take you where they may, without fearing the outcome. The more honest you are, the more clearly your soul's voice will speak to you, helping you along the path towards a life free of constant thoughts of food, regret, guilt — toward a life that is truly yours: pleasurable, exuberant, loving and joyful.

We begin with a commitment to be kind to ourselves. Our purpose is not to focus on diets, discipline and discouragement but to bring forth your innate goodness and to encourage living your life from your inner light of wholeness and love. This guidebook is not as much about your relationship with food as it is about your relationship with accepting yourself and loving yourself — and from this place, making healthy food choices.

My hope is that you will honor and integrate all you learn about yourself and embrace your life as it is right now, beginning by accepting and honoring this very moment and the beauty that surrounds you. I hope these pages will help create understanding around your relationship with food, broadening your perspective, establishing healthy nourishment for yourself and welcoming change and healing with ease and grace.

ରୁ

THE JOURNEY

Healing is a lifetime journey into our own wholeness. It is embracing what is most feared and opening to what has been closed. Healing is remembering with awareness, meaning and joy, what we have forgotten about living our lives and about being ourselves. We are not broken and we are not to blame. We have simply lost our way.

The journey of healing from unhealthy eating habits starts where you are. Any change, large or small, begins with self awareness and clear intention.

Are you willing to take a little time each day to become mindfully in touch with yourself?

Are you ready to delve, discover and transform out-dated ways of thinking and behaving into a more compassionate and truthful way of navigating life?

Are you prepared to leave behind all that is familiar and comfortable, making way for fresh, new and vibrant living?

The words of Joseph Chilton Pearce from *The Biology of Transcendence* remind us of the importance of bringing our soul and spirit to each moment and to trust the wisdom of inner knowing and of our deepest selves: *"Transcendence, the ability to rise, and go beyond limitation and restraint, is our biological birthright, built into us genetically and blocked by enculturation ... Once we have been faithful in small works by which we learn to trust the life process, larger and larger works become possible".*

CR

In addition, science has shown us that even the subtlest changes in how we think and behave will significantly change brain chemistry in a positive and healthy way. Neural integration — brain and body balance and health — is what we will achieve as an outcome of changing our behavior in even the smallest way.

If you wish for a life well lived — a life of wellness, well-being and inner tranquility — please give yourself the gift of "21 Days of Eating Mindfully".

In these pages, we will explore:

H: Hunger and Healing

E: Empathy and Emotional Eating

A: Awareness and Acceptance

L: Love and Letting Be

I: Inquiry and Intention

N: Nurture and Nourishment

G: Gratitude and Gracious Living

You will find the following 21 days to be a beginner's guide to healing your relationship with yourself: returning to love and to honoring your wholeness. And from this deep inner core, the discovery of making new and healthy choices in regards to food and eating habits from a foundation of clear intention and commitment is possible. Even more, this is a guide for loving yourself once again and allowing and encouraging your inner self to bloom and flourish with strength, faith and hope.

CR

There are three pages for each of the letters in "HEALING". Each page contains "food for thought", related mindfulness activities and points to ponder. You can choose to begin each morning with a page or end each day as you reflect back. This is simply an introduction to the principles and truths of reconnecting with yourself and beginning to look at your life in a loving, forgiving and compassionate way.

IF NOT NOW, WHEN?

Stop for a moment and ask yourself:

How would I live if I fully believed that I am whole, free and deserving of health and wellness?

Would I worry less and enjoy life more?

Would I immerse myself in the beauty and richness of life, not letting fear or uncertainty stop me from anything?

Would I eat when my body is hungry, choosing healthy foods — stopping when I feel full and truly satisfied?

How, then, would I live? And if not now, when?

When we live with the constant and unrelenting belief that we will be a better person, more lovable and happier, if we achieve something "out there" such as a lower weight, a smaller dress size or an element of control, we will never be at ease with ourselves because what we long for lies within. And when our attempts at achievement fall short of our expectations, we turn to the easiest and most trustable form of instant comfort and gratification: food.

☙

Unhealthy eating behavior is not a food issue but a relationship issue — with yourself and how well you love the person you are and have always been. On this 21 day journey we "open to" rather than "turn away from" our compulsive and disordered eating habits, allowing them to be our teachers — our guides back to our true self. As we learn to pause and listen mindfully to the voice of these compulsions, we are then able to be aware, compassionate, forgiving, loving and wise human beings. We become able to live from our core — from the center of who we are with wisdom, connection and deep love. As we transform our habit of seeking answers or solutions from somewhere outside of ourselves to trusting our own innate wisdom and knowledge, we become a healing presence for ourselves, our relationships and our world.

This 21 day journey is a guide to establishing a healthy relationship with yourself — a loving relationship with yourself — enjoying wise eating choices as a natural result and weight loss and stabilization as a natural outcome.

To embark on this journey you must do five things:

1. Leave behind all that is familiar and comfortable

2. Open to truth, compassion and forgiveness

3. Accept that you are already whole and there is nothing broken

4. Know that everyone and everything is your teacher

5. Embrace true and lasting change that comes from love, not discipline or dieting

CR

The journey also asks that you make a perceptual shift from disliking and judging who you have been to loving the possibility of who you are now and who you can become.

Welcome to *21 Days of Eating Mindfully, Your Guide to a Healthy Relationship with Yourself and Food.* May your heart guide you along the way and may the generations of women seeking and discovering their own best selves be your strength and foundation. [B1]

Hunger and Healing

"When we honor our true hunger for nourishment, there are no "good" or "bad" foods. There is no "on a diet" or "off a diet" behavior. There is nothing to feel guilty about or to regret. Our self-worth remains whole while we connect with our innate wisdom—learning to honor our body's signals."

—Lorrie Jones

We begin with hunger and healing because food and feeling better about eating habits is why most people seek help and guidance. In this section we address bodily hunger, how to recognize it and the skills involved in nourishing our bodies wisely. We also address a deeper hunger: the longing for a life of authenticity, honesty, freedom and joy. Anyone who eats or behaves compulsively is seeking a reconnection with her core self — with the person inside who is loving, innocent and blameless. Unhealthy eating, then, begins to reveal itself as an attempt to love oneself — to bring comfort, compassion, creativity or perhaps safety to a life of discipline, emotional pain and judgment.

We will learn to distinguish true hunger from a longing for something else in life by eating mindfully — a practice that breaks through every overeating or under eating experience because it requires awareness, attention and presence. As we explore mindful eating and how to incorporate this practice into our lives, we begin to cultivate the possibility of a lifestyle that encourages and honors expression of and respect for who we are.

CR

What we learn here encourages and supports mindful awareness of hunger on a physical level as well as hunger on a deep, emotional and spiritual level — and how to meet both with a loving heart. Once there is awareness there can be healing. And with awareness there is learning. Overeating or compulsive eating (and related behaviors) are not food issues but relationship issues: how we love or do not love the person we are and have always been.

Healing from unhealthy eating habits and their consequences in our lives is not about a quick fix or an overnight cure. Though "instant" might sound appealing at first, most of us long for a richer life — one with meaning, purpose, happiness and peace. Through everyday choices it is possible to reconnect to the core of our true being — and to the life we long for: one balanced and aligned with what we most treasure and enjoy.

CR

Hunger and Healing, Day 1

> "If love could speak to you about food, it would say, 'Eat when you are hungry, sweetheart, because if you don't, you won't enjoy the taste of food. And why should you do anything you don't enjoy?'"
>
> — Geneen Roth, Women, Food and God

Do you ever find yourself reaching for food when you're not hungry?

Do you eat out of: boredom, loneliness, frustration or other emotions?

If so, does it leave you satisfied or feeling guilty and unfulfilled?

Is it possible that your true hunger is for something deeper — something not related to food at all?

True hunger — the need for nourishment — is a sensation felt in the body. Hunger is experienced uniquely by each individual person. Becoming aware of your body's physical hunger is a beginning and an important step in learning to eat mindfully.

Bring mindful awareness to the sensations in your body before eating and ask yourself: am I feeling hungry? How do I know I am hungry? What signals are present for me?

As you begin to establish mindful eating habits, you may find it helpful to have guidelines to refer to. The following suggestions are meant to support you as you begin to establish awareness of hunger and mindful eating habits.

CR

- Reject the dieting mentality – no matter what it takes
- Honor your hunger – eat what your body truly wants
- Make peace with food – refuse to see it as 'the enemy'
- Eat when you are truly hungry – allow hunger to happen
- Stop eating when your body is full – regardless
- Eat without distraction
- Eat sitting down – savor
- Eat as if everyone is watching
- Cope with feelings without eating
- Honor your body, the nourishment and the experience
- Enjoy the food, the taste and be grateful

MINDFULNESS ACTIVITY

Determine your hunger signals before eating. How do you know you're hungry? Where do you feel hunger in your body? What are you hungry for?

Decide what your body wants. Imagine the texture, temperature and taste of a desired food. Imagine the approximate proportion appropriate for you, now.

JOURNAL

Before eating your next meal, pause and ask yourself the above questions. If how you nourish your body is how you feed your soul, how would you change the way you eat? What kind of meal would you plan for yourself? What habit would you let go of first?

Notice how you feel after reflecting on the questions: what sensations are present? Please write about your experience and your discoveries.

CR

"There are realities we all share, regardless of our nationality, language, or individual tastes. As we need food, so do we need emotional nourishment: love, kindness, appreciation, and support from others. We need to understand our environment and our relationship to it. We need to fulfill certain inner hungers: the need for happiness, for peace of mind, for wisdom."

—J. Donald Walters

Often we eat with distraction and haste, habitually and mindlessly. The following suggestions offer a basic set of guidelines for eating in a more mindful manner. What if you ate meals and snacks, in front of others or as if you were in the presence of others? What might you notice? Would you change any habits, knowing others were 'watching'?

MINDFULNESS ACTIVITY

- Create a lovely place setting
- Eat sitting down and in a calm place (if possible)
- Pause before eating and center yourself in the moment
- Be grateful for the food
- Eat what your body wants
- Focus on the taste, texture and temperature of the food
- Chew each bite mindfully, putting your fork down in between bites

- Eat without distractions such as TV or the newspaper
- Eat until you are satisfied, leaving food on your plate, if necessary
- Be aware of thoughts or emotions that appear

JOURNAL

Eat one meal mindfully and in silence, focusing on the above suggestions. Notice any thoughts, emotions or sensations that may be present. How are you experiencing awareness?

Please write about your experience of eating mindfully. What was new for you? What did you discover about yourself?

ℭ℞

> *"Ultimately, the most important learning about nutrition is not only about what is wise to eat, but how our relationship to food is our teacher that informs us about who we are, what we value and how it is possible to live, give and love from our deepest level of being."*
>
> —Lorrie Jones

Many times, the end of a meal is not the end of the meal. Nibbling, finishing someone else's plate, or snacking mindlessly can be a tough habit to break. Bringing mindful awareness to the ending of a meal, determine if you are satisfied or not. Listen to your body when it says "enough for now". Doing so will begin to end compulsive eating because focused awareness and mindless behavior cannot co-exist.

Transitioning from a snack or a meal can be difficult and challenging and therefore an ideal time to implement mindfulness skills. As the last bite is chewed, take a moment to breathe deeply and notice how you feel, reminding yourself you are complete for now. Then take the first step toward your next activity – again, mindfully and consciously. This is a new moment, a new beginning.

Be with this moment fully, bringing awareness to any sensations, thoughts and emotions you may be experiencing. Continue to breathe deeply....noticing. Is there "part of you" that wants to linger in the previous moments of eating? If so, what does this "part" of you need? After acknowledging the need, is it possible to move forward with 100% agreement within?

Continue to breathe deeply until you are ready to take the next step, and with complete awareness, transition from this moment to the next moment. Continuing to breathe deeply, bring a focused awareness to "now". Allow yourself fully to be in this moment....and the next....and the next. In time, you will experience a sense of ease and flow — grace and tranquility.

MINDFULNESS ACTIVITY

At the end of a meal, ask yourself: how do I feel physically? Am I satiated? How do I know this? Do I feel energized or is there another sensation present?

Notice your transition. What follows eating? Are you able to make a smooth transition to your next activity? Is your mind clear or is it clouded by thoughts related to food, eating or control issues?

JOURNAL

Allow yourself to be aware of your body, your thoughts and emotions without judging them. Notice if you feel full or still hungry, energetic or fatigued. Are any judgmental thoughts creeping in?

Notice if there was ease for you in your transition after eating a meal. Please write about your experience.

Empathy and Emotional Eating

"Emotional eating is when you eat in response to feelings rather than hunger, usually as a way to suppress or relieve negative emotions. Stress, anxiety, sadness, boredom, anger, loneliness, relationship problems and poor self-esteem can all trigger emotional eating. When emotions determine your eating habits rather than your stomach, it can quickly lead to overeating, weight gain and guilt."

—Joy Bauer

In this section, we address the need for empathy — a heartfelt understanding and compassion —as we begin to become aware of emotional eating and the damage it does to our bodies, souls and spirits. We learn that we have been trying very hard, perhaps for years, to get away from painful feelings and unwanted sensations and trying, instead, to move toward an experience of feeling good about ourselves. We have perceived ourselves as broken and in need of a cure — something or someone from the outside who can fix us. When such attempts fail we become filled with guilt, shame and despair, and often turn to food for comfort and security.

What we really long for is the ability to be fully present with ourselves, no matter what. The skill of being present in each moment, without blame or judgment, is called mindfulness. In this section, we apply the skills of mindfulness to emotions and eating. We explore eating mindfully, learning to pause and slow down — to savor each bite — and to be aware of our feelings, thoughts and sensations. Though emotions may arise, we learn ways to recognize feelings and find other ways to respond to them than overeating or eating mindlessly.

Learning to bring empathy into each eating situation will begin to illuminate the difference between "false comfort" and "true comfort" and encourage the transformation of self-destructive habits into habits of nourishment, self-respect and honor. We find it possible to move from disliking ourselves to loving ourselves — embracing all of who we are and the rich possibility of who we can become.

ೞ

Empathy and Emotional Eating, Day 4

> "When we drink tea in mindfulness, we practice coming back to the present moment to live our life right here. When our mind and our body are fully in the present moment, then the steaming cup of tea appears clearly to us. We know it is a wonderful aspect of existence. At that time, we are really in contact with the cup of tea. It is only at times like this that life is really present."
>
> —Thich Nhat Hanh

Before being able to identify emotional eating patterns, empathy and self- understanding is essential. How many times have you blamed yourself for not having more "control" or "willpower"? Often, judgment and harshness follow, leaving a path of shame and guilt. What once looked like discipline has actually been the creation of an internal dictator with a voice of fear and criticism.

We must honor ourselves and our unmet needs with empathy — as if we took a step away, and looked at our own body and soul with love and compassion. We are all products of our society, our backgrounds and our thought patterns. While we can't change the unchangeable, we can change how we view our circumstances and ultimately our lives. We always have the freedom of response: how we choose to think and behave in every situation. When we change our minds, we change every cell in our body.

MINDFULNESS ACTIVITY

Stop — be still for a few moments and look at yourself with eyes of compassion and understanding: can you see a person deserving of love, honor and respect? Can you begin to identify times when you turn to food for emotional reasons? Can you imagine eating one meal mindfully — being aware of the taste and texture of the food, chewing each bite thoroughly and pausing often to enjoy the food, stopping when you feel full and satisfied?

As you think of eating, what comes to mind? An emotion? A thought? What are some beliefs you were raised with regarding eating? For example: "You must clean your plate." How have some of these beliefs impacted your life, your habits, and how you connect or disconnect with yourself? Pause, breathe deeply, and ponder. What comes up for you?

JOURNAL

While being aware of the body, ask yourself: "What do I want to eat?" Am I hungry for nourishment or for something "deeper"? Allow an emotion or an "aha" to surface...breathe into it...write about it. With empathy, allow yourself to imagine a response other than eating.

Empathy and Emotional Eating, Day 5

> *"Each woman wants something different, yet each woman wants the same thing — to be who she truly is, to become all that she can be, and to be understood and loved for who she is."*
>
> — Lorrie Jones

To live in a healthy way, eating intuitively and loving our lives, we must acknowledge our feelings fully. Unacknowledged feelings often underlie compulsive eating for many people. A feeling or a sensation in the body is a natural "primary" experience. When we allow thoughts, opinions and judgments to invade and be believable, we create a secondary experience called a "reaction" — a combination of an emotion and a thought form.

As we are learning, in order to become in touch with hunger and fullness cues and to truly know what the body is craving, it is important to be mindful while eating. Using our senses is a profound way to "listen" to our bodies while eating. Many of us are rushing around and eating food on the run. Eating in this manner, most of us do not pay attention to hunger and fullness cues — nor to the taste, texture, sight and smell of the food. Staying fully aware of these aspects of food will enhance the experience of eating, and more enjoyment and satisfaction will be experienced.

Asking questions and being curious and mindful during mealtimes is beneficial for anyone wanting to become a more intuitive eater. Awareness is such an important component of change. Without awareness we may find it impossible to become an intuitive eater and to move beyond the diet mentality.

If you know you are an emotional eater, the following skill can be very helpful. Donald Altman, a mindfulness teacher, suggests **STOP**: stopping for mindfulness.

> **S:** Select: Be purposeful in deciding what to eat and how much
>
> **T:** Taste: Enjoy each bite and taste the deliciousness. Chew slowly and deliberately...pausing between bites
>
> **O:** Observe: notice everything about this bite, including thoughts and feelings
>
> **P:** Pause in the midst of a bite...notice. Continue chewing and pause again at the end of the bite. Notice: Are you hungry for more?

Checking in throughout the meal can also help us to be mindful while eating. Ask questions such as:

- Where is my hunger or fullness level?
- Am I enjoying this food?
- What would make my eating experience more pleasurable in this moment?
- Would I rather be eating something else?
- Am I staying present while I am eating, or is my mind wandering?
- What external events influenced my food choices today?
- How can I reconnect to the internal signals my body is giving me?

MINDFULNESS ACTIVITY

Eat one meal mindfully, incorporating "STOP". Was it difficult to eat slowly, savoring every bite? Was it calming to eat slowly? What was your experience? Were you able to notice thoughts and emotions and the tendency to "react"?

JOURNAL

Did the STOP method help you practice mindfulness of the meal? Are you willing to make this a mealtime habit? Why or why not? How will you remember to use this method with future eating?

Empathy and Emotional Eating, Day 6

> *"The way you eat is inseparable from your core beliefs about being alive."*
>
> —Geneen Roth, Women, Food and God

How we eat is how we live: how we honor ourselves or destroy ourselves, how we create or negate health, how we blame and chastise ourselves or forgive, love and honor ourselves. Looking honestly at your life, how might your relationship with food be a mirror for your life? What are your deepest beliefs and how do they show up on your plate? Do you turn to food for comfort, sweetness or reassurance?

When we reach for food excessively, often something within wants to emerge. With careful attention, painful issues with food and eating, met in non-violent, compassionate ways, can illuminate the areas in need of healing.

What might it take for you to change your approach to food and eating? Could your very compulsions be a doorway to learning and a bridge from a life of powerlessness to one of choice and strength?

Let's take a look at reacting versus responding. Reacting is a knee-jerk experience: before we know it, we are taking action in a mindless fashion. Responding, however, is a conscious act and a choice to be fully present to what's happening. With responding, we suspend expectation and judgment. There is no question that responding takes more effort. Responding also asks us to grow as a person which can be frightening. Yet, as we grow, we become more mature — more centered, focused and compassionate. Notice how often you react instead of respond. What kinds of things are you reactive to? Begin to notice your tender spots and be curious as to what could be the "issue" for you. Is it possible to bring compassion and empathy to yourself and begin to change your ways?

When we stop an automatic behavior, when we create a pause between a thought and the action or speech that usually follows, we are wedging open the door to a prison made of hundreds of old habit patterns, conditioned over time. When these old habits show themselves, we have choice. And with wise choice, our recovery and healing moves forward.

Gregory Kramer, author of *Insight Dialogue: The Interpersonal Path to Freedom* suggests the following: first of all, pause — then relax and be open, listen deeply and speak the truth. When leading workshops, he also guides participants to "trust emergence", understanding that impermanence is always at play and nothing ever stays the same. Dr. Kramer's suggestions could be a "guide for responding". Take a few minutes and commit to memory: *pause, relax, open, trust emergence, listen deeply and speak the truth.*

The applications of responding versus reacting are numerous. One of the most powerful uses of "pause, relax, open, trust emergence, listen deeply and speak the truth" is with emotional eating. Bringing this level of awareness to the "reaction" of eating from emotional pressures can be remarkably healing.

Developing the practice of pausing, in itself, invites awareness — and with awareness can come wise choice. And with wise choice, over time, the body will return to health.

CR

MINDFULNESS ACTIVITY

When strong emotions arise — anger, frustration, anxiety or confusion — you may turn to food for comfort. How do your moods affect your eating habits? Do you choose certain foods for certain moods? What patterns do you notice? Is it possible to feel your feelings, embrace and "live them" without attaching a story line to them? Reflect on any connections you discover between your moods and your eating habits. Do you tend to eat in response to certain situations? What are "triggers" for you? Can you stop and breathe first — even for a moment? What might be asking for room to emerge in your life? Can you imagine your struggles with food and eating being doorways to learning and growth?

JOURNAL

Take a moment to compassionately reflect upon your discoveries from the above questions. How might you integrate what you have learned into your current habits? Are you ready to give up the familiar pattern of turning to food for comfort and then drowning in guilt? Would it be possible to pause, breathe and "wait out" an emotion that normally leads to eating? What happens to the emotion? Is it possible to imagine a feeling being like a cloud that passes by? Can you let it "be" and continue to breathe? Please write about doorways and bridges in your life. Is your heart open to loving yourself fully?

CR

Awareness and Acceptance

"Wherever you are is the entry point."

—Kabir

Bringing mindful awareness and loving acceptance to your body and to your life will change your entire relationship with food. You will begin to live each day in acceptance of who you are and what you truly need. You will begin to love yourself, seeing clearly that you are blameless and unbroken.

In this section we explore what it means to become aware and the importance of pausing and embracing each moment. Rather than continuing a life of partial attention or one of "automatic pilot", we learn to bring a mindful awareness to our days, our moments, and our behavior. All healing begins with awareness. Becoming aware of thoughts, opinions and judgments around food and eating will change your life forever. When we begin to understand what drives us to eat when we are not hungry and how we blame ourselves for being too full, punishing ourselves with guilt and remorse, we hold the key to our true self — the person who dwells within wanting authentic expression, love and acceptance.

In childhood we are taught many things yet we are not taught to be ok with ourselves — to accept and love ourselves as we are. So, long ago, we became on-going "projects" to improve upon and fix in some way, focusing on what must change rather than meeting ourselves from within and loving the person we find there. It is possible to open our hearts once again and through forgiveness and mercy, begin to heal. Until we live in full acceptance of ourselves and love ourselves from the inside out, the unwanted habits and the undesirable weight will remain.

In this section, we learn to quiet ourselves and our minds and listen to our bodies. We explore love and living with life's challenges — and the practice of mindfulness. Healing is dependent upon awareness and self-acceptance. Our purpose is to become aware and curious, cultivating mindfulness, tenderness and love. It is awareness and acceptance, not deprivation and discipline, that nurture healthy habits. Presence — not denial or escape — changes perspective, inviting us to respond to life rather than react to it. When we honor our bodies with awareness and acceptance, we begin to fully reclaim our feelings, our experiences and our lives.

Awareness and Acceptance, Day 7

> *"The secret of health for both mind and body is not to mourn for the past, not to worry about the future, and not to anticipate troubles, but to live in the present moment wisely and earnestly."*
>
> —Buddha

The first step toward being a mindful eater is to become aware of each moment, by bringing non-judgmental curiosity, openness and acceptance to whatever is arising. This is sometimes easier said than done! Awareness is often clouded by the many "should do" and "must do" messages often bombarding our present moment and demanding priority. Becoming mindfully aware, moment to moment, invites us to re-focus our attention and awareness. We look with inquiry at what is actually "here", including the assumptions and opinions we continually make.

As we have said, all healing begins with awareness. Mindful awareness is the key to well-being and overall mental and emotional health. Focused awareness activates specific circuits of the brain, which promote balance and healthy integration in our lives. Becoming aware of your own thought world around food and shifting any stressful and ineffective behaviors regarding nourishment and eating habits will change your life forever. When you begin to understand what prompts you to eat when you are not hungry, you hold the ticket to the center of your soul, to your true self. When you accept with compassion what is hidden and shameful, the path to healing appears. Ready to end the familiar turmoil of endless dieting and attempts at control?

CR

Find a quiet, comfortable place to sit. Try keeping your back straight and gently supported, with your shoulder blades slightly dropped and your chin gently tucked toward your chest. Take three, slow easy deep breaths to relax and let go of whatever burdens you are carrying. Let your eyelids gently close. Bring your attention to your breathing. Pay attention to where you notice your breathing most strongly. Perhaps it's the nostrils...perhaps the abdomen...simply notice. Now, discover when you feel your breath more strongly – when you exhale or when you inhale. Let your body breathe for you and simply pay attention to the air in your nose each time you inhale and exhale, one breath after another. If your mind wanders away from the sensation of the breath, no worries. Gently return to the feeling of your in-breath and out-breath at the nostrils any time you notice your mind has wandered. After about 15 minutes, gently and slowly open your eyes. Savor the stillness of the moment before moving on.

MINDFULNESS ACTIVITY

Whatever your journey, you must start where you are. Ask yourself: what am I aware of right now? Where do I experience this awareness in my body? What do I taste, smell, hear, feel or see? What thoughts are present? Is there a pattern? Is my relationship with food a possible gift opening me to living a life of health and healing?

JOURNAL

Describe your experience. Was it easy or difficult for you to be still and notice? What thoughts emerged? Did emotion follow these thoughts? Can you name or describe them? Are you open to accepting your food struggles as a blessing?

CR

Awareness and Acceptance, Day 8

> *"When we welcome what we most want to avoid, we contact a part of ourselves that is fresh and alive."*
>
> — Geneen Roth, Women, Food and God

Bringing mindful awareness and attention to our body can change our entire relationship with food and eating — and, of course, with ourselves. Without mindfully attending to our bodies, we may become so busy in our daily lives that we lose touch with how to eat — with our hunger and our intuitive sense of what to eat at the time. We lose touch with ourselves and what we truly want for our lives.

In healing mindfully, we direct a compassionate and loving attention to the deepest parts of our pain and the innermost depth of our wounds. This is where healing occurs. When we honor our bodies with our attention, we begin to reclaim our feelings, our experiences and our lives. When we open to what has been closed or denied, we lessen the desire for overeating or under-eating.

MINDFULNESS ACTIVITY

Sit quietly and ask: what is my body saying to me right now? Is there a particular part of me that is asking for a more loving attention? Write about one area wanting compassionate acceptance: how have I been ignoring this part of me? How might I begin to accept this part? Ask yourself: am I willing to stop the struggle? Ask yourself: how can I love myself more?

JOURNAL

Allow yourself to become still and aware of your body, your sensations, and your thoughts without judging them. Please write about your experience and your discoveries.

Practice listening to your body and bringing a loving and compassionate presence to each moment. Is there a part of your life, body or emotions that is disconnected or feels abandoned? Can you cherish and bring a healing presence to this part?

> *"...There is no need to search...Release your struggle, let go of your mind, throw away your concerns, and relax into the world. No need to resist life. Open your eyes and see that you are far more than you think. You are already free."*
>
> —*Dan Millman, No Ordinary Moments*

Acceptance is a form of wisdom, an act of love. Acceptance does not mean we have to like something or become a doormat in our lives. Rather, acceptance means we simply "let be" what is here, now. We are simply acknowledging what exists without reacting with judgment or opinion. Living with awareness and acceptance means becoming all that we are and allowing that self to flourish and bloom. This is a matter of self-discovery rather than becoming something or someone else.

As Dan Millman suggests, there is no need to search or struggle. If you are ready to be true to yourself, your way back to truth is on your plate. Once you accept who you are — now, right now — and honor all past behaviors as choices made for very good reasons at the time, you are free. And it becomes more important to lose weight from wholeness than from fear — from self-love than from self-hate.

MINDFULNESS ACTIVITY

Bring to mind something in your life that is difficult for you to accept. Pause, breathe and open, as best, to this presence. Ask yourself: what is difficult about this issue? Is there a gift, a positive intention, to it? What do you see as the primary lesson of this "difficult" situation? Is it possible to taste freedom in the midst of feeling trapped?

JOURNAL

Sit quietly, allowing yourself to become calm and receptive. Think of a difficulty you are currently facing

Notice how this difficulty is affecting your body. Now ask yourself: how have I treated this difficulty so far? How have I suffered from my own response? What am I being asked to let go of? What lesson might be present for me? What is the possible gift in this situation? Please record your discoveries.

CR

Love and Letting Be

> *"The easiest way to work on letting go and letting be is to notice your tendency to want things to be different from what they are and to practice giving up that strong preference. The Third Chinese Patriarch of Zen sang, 'The Way is not difficult for those who have few preferences'."*

—*Lama Surya Das*

In this section, we take a look at the true elements of healing unwanted eating habits and the disturbing and blaming thoughts that accompany compulsive behavior. To heal, we must learn to love in every situation. We are looking at the heart and soul of what is required in order to heal from unwanted and out of control eating habits.

Love is accepting, affirming and honoring. It is patient and deeply understanding. Love sees what is without any demand to change it. Loving means choosing to be in unconditional acceptance and support of who we are and of what is happening at all times, with no exceptions. It means getting to know, love and accept the part of us that overeats.

The purpose of this section is to support healing the relationship between the part of you that nourishes yourself wisely and the part of you that eats in a less than healthy way. These are two "beings" within the whole of who you are and they both deserve love, honor and deep respect. We over eat, under eat or over control for very good reasons.

The lesson in loving and letting be is learning to embrace, not deny, the perceived "imperfect" you — the struggling you — who is a product of pain, fear and betrayal on many levels. This being needs love, not discipline, to heal. And it is a deep and abiding love that will soothe, reassure and support the wholeness and expression of this healthy self. Until we live in full acceptance of ourselves and love ourselves from the inside out, unwanted habits will rule, unhealthy weight will remain and undesirable controlling behavior will reign.

Our struggles with weight issues are masquerading on a body level but are problems whose solution can only be found on a spiritual level — from the inner core of our being. The purpose, therefore, is to accept and "let be" all that is in our lives right now and begin to let love — forgiveness, compassion and kindness — lead us into our wholeness and goodness.

CR

Love and Letting Be, Day 10

> *"If your heart is pure, then all things in your world are pure....then the moon and flowers will guide you along the way."*
>
> — Ryokan

In undertaking any new learning or new journey, we must ask ourselves: "does this path have heart?" And more importantly, "is my heart connected with my path?" No one can define for us what our path is, as each person's path is unique. Instead we must ask ourselves and then listen, with awareness and acceptance, to our answers. We must look honestly at the life we have chosen so far and notice where we put our time, our energy, our creativity and our love. Does the life I am choosing reflect my deepest and truest values?

To live our path with heart and love allows the preciousness of life to fill us. Too easily we forget our deepest intentions — yet most people, myself included, who have faced death's door, do not overly concern ourselves with money in the bank or a list of accomplishments. Rather, we ask ourselves: "Did I love well?" And we know that being loved in return is our greatest gift.

Freedom from compulsions is not something we must create. It is about being fully who we are and being committed to loving in every situation. The longing for love and happiness is underneath all of our wishing and reaching. Often we look in all the wrong places — the refrigerator being one of many dead ends. What we long for we already possess. We don't really need more or require our lives to be different in order to be fulfilled and happy. We possess the ability to love all of life and honor the sacredness of each person's journey, especially our own.

MINDFULNESS ACTIVITY

Ask yourself: does my life reflect my deepest values? Am I able to say, "Yes, I love well"? Am I willing to love myself, right now, the way I am? If not, why and what will it take? Can you think of a specific habit that needs your love and understanding? Is it possible to bring love – forgiveness, compassion, kindness – to whatever situation is present for you?

Start with sitting quietly and let your body be at rest. As best, let go of plans and future thinking. Say to yourself: "May I be filled with loving and kindness". Continue to sit quietly, repeating these words silently. Begin to allow your life to illuminate itself, breathing into all of "what is". Gently and as you are ready, give thanks for all that is in your life – tenderly letting go of striving....of wanting things to be different in order to be happier.

JOURNAL

What did you discover about yourself? What are some of your deepest values? What is one habit that is in need of your acceptance, love and understanding? Are you able to begin to give thanks for all that is in your life? Please write about your experiences.

Loving and Letting Be, Day 11

> "Loving yourself requires us to believe in and stay loyal to something no one else can see...our own self worth."
>
> —Mark Nepo

There can be no true path with heart without loving-kindness. Mindfulness is above all a loving embrace of the moment — this moment, not a different moment wished for or longed for. The wisdom to love and the courage to do so are within us. We simply forget. We, instead, believe that love exists outside of us, waiting to be discovered or earned. It's time to wake up, is it not? Awakening your heart nurtures a natural, graceful and expansive ability to love in every situation. And only love heals.

The following meditation is called a "loving-kindness meditation". Loving-kindness is an "acquired skill". Many of us find this meditation awkward at first. This is because most of us have an expectation for how we "should" feel during a meditation. Yet as Sharon Salzberg reminds us: *"loving-kindness meditation works even if you don't feel a thing!"*

MINDFULNESS ACTIVITY

Please set aside 20 minutes for the purpose of giving yourself loving attention. Sit in a comfortable position, reasonably upright and relaxed. Close your eyes and bring your attention to the heart region of your body. Now take three slow, easy breaths from the heart. Remember that every living being wants to live peacefully and happily.

Connect with your breath: *"Just as all beings wish to be happy and free from suffering, may I be happy and free from suffering."* Let yourself feel the warmth of this loving attention.

Repeat, silently, the following phrases:

> *May I be safe*
>
> *May I be happy*
>
> *May I be healthy*
>
> *May I live with ease*

Take your time and with an open heart, savor the meaning of these words. When you notice that your mind has wandered (as it will), simply repeat the phrases again. Whenever you feel lost, return to the phrases and repeat them. Let this exercise be easy. Don't try too hard. Loving-kindness is the most natural thing in the world. Distractions will always arise, and when you notice them, let them go on by and return to the phrases. Sit with yourself as if you would sit with a dear friend who is ill; you may not cure the illness but you will impart the kindness the friend deserves. Gently open your eyes. Is there a shift of awareness? Do you believe you deserve kindness, wellness and peace?

JOURNAL

Before loving others, we must first love ourselves. Did you find this activity difficult? Easy? Do you find it difficult to love yourself? Please write about your experience.

CR

Loving and Letting Be, Day 12

"Loving ourselves opens us to truly knowing ourselves as part of a matrix of existence, inextricably connected to the boundlessness of life. When we keep opening past any version of who we are that is crafted by others, when we see that we are far bigger than the person that is delineated by family or cultural expectations, we realize that we are capable of so much more than we usually dare to imagine. In this spirit the poet Walt Whitman wrote, I am larger, better than I thought; I did not know I held so much goodness."

—Sharon Salzberg, *The Force of Kindness*

Cultivating the idea of letting go as a part of loving ourselves is essential to practicing mindfulness of food and eating. As we begin to pay attention to our experience, we instantly find that certain thoughts and feelings are present and, in fact, seem to repeat themselves as if they are true. If the thoughts are "pleasant", we tend to hang onto them. If they are, instead, "unpleasant", we tend to avoid them or try to push them away or deny their existence. Sometimes the desire to lose weight is more deeply a desire to destroy disruptive thoughts bombarding the mind.

First of all, mindfulness asks us to let these thoughts, and often feelings following the thoughts, be present and to reveal themselves. We simply observe, impartially. Then we practice "letting go" of the thoughts, allowing them to float on by like clouds in the sky. Letting go is a way of "letting be" — of accepting things just as they are, moment to moment, without attaching our thinking, such as judgment, to anything.

MINDFULNESS ACTIVITY

Sit quietly and observe the breath. Where do you feel the breath? In the nostrils? In the throat? Allowing breathing to continue calmly, pay attention to thoughts. Is there a pattern to thoughts? Do they have a certain quality? Are you able to return awareness to the breath each time thoughts wander? Are you able to gently begin to release thoughts - letting them "be", noticing the impermanence of a thought – how it shifts and changes, eventually disappearing?

JOURNAL

What did you notice about the breath? How do you feel now? Did you feel bombarded by thoughts? Did they have urgency to them? Perhaps your thoughts were kind in nature. What did you notice? Was it possible for you to be aware of a thought being just that: a thought? Write about building the "muscle" of bringing attention back to the present each time it wanders off.

CR

Inquiry and Intention

"Our intention creates our reality."

—Wayne Dyer

As we continue to discover and learn about ourselves, it becomes time to do an assessment of "now": to look at things as they truly are. Inquiry is our method for asking and discovering what is present and what is true. In this section we inquire into our relationship with ourselves. We explore intention and commitment and learn that until there is loyalty to oneself in all ways there cannot be loyalty to a healthy eating pattern. Until we inquire into our relationship with who we are and define and commit to what we want for ourselves, our relationship with food remains untamed. Inquiry is how we ask and learn.

Our purpose is to cultivate curiosity about ourselves and our lives. Acceptance and "letting be" invites us to stop striving for results and to start meeting our lives as they are. The quality of inquiry is directly related to the depth of our healing. Cultivating inquiry, curiosity and intentional living provides the understanding and information we need to return to "being" and the encouragement and clarity we need to live an extraordinary life. Intention is how we look at the past, the present and the future and how we envision and put into place the life we desire.

In this section of inquiry and intention, we delve, discover and deconstruct old and harmful ways of thinking and believing. We become able to undo and let go of outdated and dysfunctional ideas about ourselves, allowing and prompting us to change our story. We are then able to be fully present with wonder, joy and amazement — available to us in each moment. We are able to live by intention and in full engagement with life again, no matter what our history or present circumstance reveals.

All change begins with where we are right now. Mindfulness is deliberately paying attention, being fully aware of what is happening inside yourself – in your mind, heart and body – and outside yourself, in your environment. Mindfulness is awareness without judgment or criticism. In mindful eating we are not comparing or judging. We are simply being a witness to the many sensations, thoughts and emotions that come up around eating. This is done is an aware way, warmed with kindness and curiosity.

ॐ

Inquiry and Intention, Day 13

> "As one may bring himself to believe almost anything he is inclined to believe, it makes all the difference whether we begin or end with the inquiry, "What is truth?"
>
> — Richard Whately

Inquiry, I have come to believe, asks four questions of us:

1. *Am I showing up fully?*
2. *Am I paying attention (to what has heart and meaning)?*
3. *Am I open to outcome or am I attached to outcome?*
4. *Am I telling my truth without blame or judgment?*

Of course, there are many ways of inquiry — of asking truthful questions of ourselves and of our lives. From many years of experience and learning, I have embraced the above four questions, adapted from Angeles Arrien and *The Four-Fold Way*. Through the years and no matter the circumstance, these questions are timeless and guide me on my way.

Perhaps the best way to begin a mindful and courageous self-inquiry is to determine what you envision for your life by looking at your present situation. How have your responses to life's challenges shaped your existence? Can you contact the place of wholeness inside of you? Do you believe this person is worthy of respect? What is her vision — her hopes and dreams for herself?

Setting an intention will assist you in taking greater control of your life and of your healing. Setting an intention directs the mind by having a purpose and a plan. When you put action behind your intention, the results are powerful.

Try to set a daily intention, such as: "I live my life in a relaxed manner" or a more specific intention, such as: "I choose to take 30 minutes this morning to breathe deeply while sitting in silence." You will want to be clear about what you intend to do and to write it down. If possible, share your intention with a loved one or a good friend as an accountability step. Next, do something to demonstrate your commitment to your intention. And finally, acknowledge your action and continue on your path.

The following are a few additional points to keep in mind when setting any healing intention:

> *Only love heals*
> *Healing the mind will heal the body*
> *Your teacher resides in your pain*
> *Your despair is your greatest gift*
> *Always be prepared for transformation*
> *All of life is an opportunity for learning*

To heal you must:

> *Be present*
> *Surrender all that is familiar and comfortable*
> *Welcome what you most despise*
> *Trust that everything is a lesson*
> *Know everyone is your teacher*
> *Commit to loving in every situation*
> *Follow what has heart and meaning*
> *Accept your wholeness now – not 'after' or 'when'*

CR

Be truthful without blame or judgment

Be open to outcome, not attached to an expectation

Accept that all you need is within

MINDFULNESS ACTIVITY

Are you showing up fully in your life? Where is there strength? Where have you given away your power? Does your path in life have heart and meaning? Can you say "yes", especially in the tough times? Are you aware of attachment in your life? For example, what is your story? How do you know it is true? Could you be more open in your life and less attached to a certain outcome? Please sit quietly and practice setting a healing intention, remembering only love heals. What will you commit to? How will you keep this commitment?

JOURNAL

Please answer the questions above allowing your responses to deepen as you write. Then find words to express one healing intention: as a beginning point, what do you commit to and how will you keep your promise to yourself? Think about asking a family member or a trusted friend to support you in staying true to your healing intention. Please write about your experiences.

Inquiry and Intention, Day 14

"Grant that I may be given appropriate difficulties and sufferings on this journey so that my heart may be truly awakened and my practice of liberation and universal compassion may be truly fulfilled."

—*Tibetan prayer*

Often from our perceived weaknesses we can learn a new way. It is the bandaged place that lets the light in. Our teacher resides in the places of our struggles and vulnerability — where we believe we have lost our way. These places ask for surrender, for letting go, so the new can emerge. Some say compulsive eating is a deep longing to dwell in the place that is already whole and wanting emergence.

The richness of wisdom, peace and wholeness lies within each of us and within our difficulties. The doorway to mindful eating is in the midst of our current challenge with food. Rather than changing your relationship with food, try changing your relationship with yourself (in relationship to food and your health):

- Put your health on "priority" status
- Define your vision for yourself
- Align your thoughts, beliefs and actions
- Determine the steps toward this vision: this will create the structure needed
- Look inside yourself and imagine expanding...opening to possibility
- Challenge every assumption you make

- Notice judgments and critical thoughts
- How will achieving your vision impact your life and the lives of others involved?
- Commit and remain true to your word

MINDFULNESS ACTIVITY

What do I dislike about myself...my body? What was my worst day of eating or not eating? How do I define my struggle with food at this time? What if I changed my story to one of letting go of struggle? What if I gave up the effort to constantly fix myself? What gifts or teachings are present for me?

JOURNAL

Answer the above questions without blame or judgment — can you? Where do you find yourself resisting change? With compassion and kindness, imagine how each stumbling block could be a gift. If you returned to yourself, what might you find? How might you live? Please write about this.

Inquiry and Intention, Day 15

"And did you get what you wanted from this life, even so?

I did.

And what did you want?

To call myself beloved,

to feel myself beloved on the earth."

— Raymond Carver

So tell me: what do you want from the rest of your life? Are you willing to explore deeply, take a risk and leave your comfort zone? Start with a small intention, such as taking 10 minutes for yourself each morning to simply breathe deeply and greet the day — before doing anything else. Or you may prefer to look at the "big picture" and define categories of general intention setting such as "I want my life to be colorful and full of meaning". Then begin to break down what such intentions mean to you and how you may want to begin your step-by-step approach.

As you find your way to a clearly intentional life, you may feel more alive and robust. You may feel calmer and more centered. You will find yourself at choice, eliminating the need to blame or find excuses. Instead, you will be on your way to living a life of purpose, vision and love. Commitment to oneself and one's life must be 100% or self-sabotaging behaviors will emerge. To commit fully, you must take action daily: recognize thoughts fully (as thoughts, not truth); forgive mistakes; believe in your dreams and keep them clear in your mind. And always be kind to yourself.

CR

MINDFULNESS ACTIVITY

What is your vision for your life? What are your highest values? How might you create awareness of intention daily? Weekly? Yearly? Are you willing to take a little time for a collage or "vision board" by beginning to collect pictures or symbols that illustrate how you envision living your very best life? Does the thought of defining your dreams create anxiety? Does the thought of defining your dreams create joy? What is your experience?

JOURNAL

Please write about intentional living — what does this mean to you? How might you create the life you truly want? Do you doubt your deservedness? How might such a life serve you and serve others? Can you create an effective way to remind yourself daily of your intention or intentions?[2]

Nurture and Nourishment

"You gotta imagine what's never been....come on, don't mess up your time to live."

—Sue Monk Kidd, the Secret Life of Bees

While most of us know what is healthy to eat, many of us, especially in the U.S., are facing obesity. How can this be when we have all the facts we need to choose healthy eating habits? Is it possible the answers to a life free of excess weight and unwanted eating habits lie somewhere other than in information?

In this section, we address the challenge that is much deeper than what we choose to eat or not eat or how much we weigh or what size we are. From what we have learned so far, the true problem does not originate on a physical level. Though healthy nourishment is important to wellness and well-being, reaching the heart of the matter is what will bring healing and healthy living. Therefore, we examine why we eat as well as what we eat. Healing will not happen on a purely physical level. We must go deeper to find solution.

Learning to nurture ourselves is the key to learning how to truly nourish our bodies as well as our spirits. Many times we exhaust our resources of time and energy by caring for others at the expense of our own well-being. And many times we turn to the instant comfort of food for emotional support or pleasure. Our goal is to illuminate our need for deep nourishment — a caring for ourselves that does not involve eating — and begin to learn ways of meeting this need. In this section we address nurture and the need for self-care. We also review basic guidelines for healthy

CR

nourishment and eating habits, establishing the beginnings of lasting change.

Again, there can be no effective personal nurture and no establishment of healthy eating without first accepting, acknowledging and fully honoring who we are and why we eat in ways that are destructive and harmful. Clearly, dieting and the restrictions of discipline-based control are harmful and deeply disrespectful acts. No wonder we feel wounded and beaten down most of the time. Only love heals. This means we stop where we are — pausing on a continual basis and bringing our focus and attention to the present moment. We breathe in and we breathe out. And with each breath, we allow compassion, forgiveness and kindness to permeate every cell of our body. We ask "what is my lesson here?" and then we listen deeply. With acceptance and honor, we learn and grow. With tenderness and a kind heart, we let love heal — as many times a day or night as it takes until we would never consider doing anything that is not in our own best interest.

Nurture and Nourishment, Day 16

> *"Your relationship with food, no matter how conflicted, is the doorway to freedom."*
>
> —Geneen Roth, Women, Food and God

In today's world many, if not most, of us know what foods and nutrients are healthy to eat and what eating habits contribute to a well nourished body. In the past two decades, we have been saturated with information about diet and eating habits. Yet one of the major health problems in the United States is obesity — and it is on the rise. If more information were needed, wouldn't we all be slender and fit?

For most of us, the challenge is much deeper than what we put on our plate. Mindless eating represents the surface of another problem needing to be addressed. Our eating habits are messages — clues leading us to the heart of the matter. When we ignore these messages, we sever our only connection between our body and our mind.

Sensations and emotions are a complex combination of feelings and bodily experiences. If you are attentive and aware of these cues, your eating will be healthy and mindful. Yet changing your relationship with food is not always easy — a profound commitment is called for and an inner discipline is required. Only by being aware of how you relate to food will it be possible to change behaviors such as mindless eating.

CR

The *Dietary Guidelines for Americans, 2010*, released on January 31, 2011, emphasize three major goals for Americans:

- Balance calories with physical activity to manage weight
- Consume more of certain foods and nutrients such as fruits, vegetables, whole grains, fat-free and low-fat dairy products, and seafood
- Consume fewer foods with sodium (salt), saturated fats, trans fats, cholesterol, added sugars, and refined grains

MINDFULNESS ACTIVITY

Let's begin with a review of the basic guidelines for healthy nourishment. Ask yourself:

Do I eat a variety of foods?

Am I choosing a diet low in fat, saturated fat and cholesterol?

Do I eat plenty of vegetables, fruits and whole grains?

Do I use sugar and salt in moderation?

Do I drink coffee, soft drinks and alcoholic beverages in moderation?

Do I drink plenty of water to remain hydrated?

JOURNAL

For each question above, write "yes" or "no". With a non-judgmental attitude, identify areas asking for improvement. If you are willing, commit to taking one small step toward health in each area, each day.[3]

Nurture and Nourishment, Day 17

> *"It is not the easy or convenient life for which I search ... but life lived to the edge of all my possibilities."*
>
> *—Mary Anne Radmacher-Hershey*

Now that we've reviewed the basic guidelines of healthy nourishment, let's look at what happens when our eating habits sabotage us. Do you over-eat, under-eat or deprive yourself? Do you believe that a diet or an eating plan is your only answer? Are you at the mercy of your emotions, thoughts and desires? Do you believe by having a different body you'll have a different life? There is one thing I know for sure: *diets do not work* and there's no possibility for understanding and healing if we continually deprive and shame ourselves. Only love heals.

Healthy change occurs at the unseen levels first. This requires faith and trust. Lasting transformation requires a spirit of inquiry, a compassionate understanding of oneself and an openness to discovery. We eat the way we do for very good reasons. It is essential to open our hearts to this. It is also essential to bring awareness and mindfulness to our present situation rather than judgment and criticism. We become an impartial witness to our thoughts and habits. When truth is illuminated mindfully, out-of-control behaviors lessen. Within a compassionate heart, we find our way back to ourselves.

Freedom from worry and constant food control is not a diet to go on but a state of being – a state of knowing who you are and being fully present to this moment. It is embracing the life you

CR

have right now, as the person you are, and knowing what sustains you — what brings you peace, joy and love. Freedom is about having the life you want by being present to the life you have now — not the life you must create.

The need for nurturance is a genuine human need. To meet this unmet need with willpower is futile. Only when we heal the wound of feeling separate and accept and love ourselves without judgment does the need for external nurturance gradually diminish. And in the realm of eating, without willpower, without denial or self-control, without the need for should and should nots, your relationship with yourself in the face of food will change and naturally correct itself.

So trust in yourself, have faith in your abilities and focus on the beauty of each new day. Ultimately you will be able to create balance, serenity and health in body, mind and spirit.

MINDFULNESS ACTIVITY

Are you dieting, restricting or controlling how you eat right now? Are any foods considered taboo or "trigger foods"? Do you believe your life will be different — wonderful, better, sexier — if you lose weight or wear a certain dress size?

Pausing and being still: observe your thoughts and feelings about food and eating: do you ever find yourself overwhelmed or exhausted — giving all of your time away to others? Is food used as a comfort — rather than choosing a healthier alternative?

What are some healthy ways you nurture yourself? Can you imagine a life of freedom from worry and thoughts of food issues?

JOURNAL

Take time to meditate mindfully, noticing patterns of thinking and the way your mind concocts stories, judgments and opinions. Practice letting the thoughts go on by, returning to yourself.

Meditate on nurture — let your need for self-care emerge. Breathe deeply, acknowledging the information you receive. Can you envision caring for yourself without using food for comfort?

Please write about what is occurring for you, what habits you notice and what challenges are present? What are you truly hungry for? What are your beliefs about food and eating? Are these beliefs true or a story you tell yourself?

Nurture and Nourishment, Day 18

> *"If you can listen to the wisdom of your body, love this flesh and bone, dedicate yourself to its mystery, you may one day find yourself smiling from your mirror."*
>
> —Marion Woodman, Coming Home to Myself

The way we eat or don't eat is an attempt to express a part of ourselves that is hidden. I believe the part wanting attention is the innermost sanctuary of our self, of our soul. If so, we must turn toward this part, not numb ourselves with food and run or push down or deny. When we stop, pause, become aware and welcome all parts of ourselves, we begin our healing journey. As the compassionate and spiritual teacher, Jack Kornfield, states in *A Path With Heart*: "...it is the imperfect that is in need of our love". Only kindness will heal the wounds, the pain and the loneliness of having been at war with ourselves and our bodies for so long.

If you are someone who has relied on food, in some way, for emotional support, comfort or denial, please know there is hope for you. In fact, the world is offering itself to you, right here, right now. The treasure — life itself with all of its blessings — is waiting for you. You must simply open the door. It is the doorway to freedom: to enjoying food as nourishment for your body and to being free of the burdens, the shame and the disappointments of all that has strewn your path with pain and despair. This is the doorway to yourself as you truly are, to your essence, to your beauty — from hating who you perceive you have been to loving the true you who is emerging.

Embracing an optimistic perspective has been proven to improve your mood, self-esteem and overall happiness. Optimism also lowers depression and anger. Be selective; focus on the positive events in the past and begin to "reframe" the less than desirable events. See each moment as a new beginning and look to the future in terms of what can be done instead of what can't happen or seems impossible. Can a threat be a challenge and a problem an opportunity for growth?

MINDFULNESS ACTIVITY

Picture a doorway, let the image come to you: what is beyond the doorway? Can you describe what you see, in your mind's eye? Is there something in the way of you opening the door? What is stopping you? What obstacles appear in your mind's eye? What is the gift in each obstacle? How can the obstacle become a strength for you on your journey? Now open the door and walk slowly and gracefully through the doorway: what is there (here)? Can you describe the "place" with your five senses?

JOURNAL

What did you find on the other side of the door? Please write about this. Can you define your obstacles? Are you able to cultivate these perceived obstacles and allow strengths or gifts to emerge? Please write about what you have discovered about yourself.

CR

Gratitude and Gracious Living

"And today you know that's good enough for me. Breathin' in and out's a blessing can't you see. Today's the first day of the rest of my life."

—Dave Matthews, I'm Alive

In the last of our lessons, we open to gratitude and living a gracious life. I remember, long ago, first being introduced to the concept of being grateful — for everything. Living in constant gratitude didn't come easily for me as I was raised to judge life as good or bad, events as right or wrong and my endeavors as successes or failures. My world was black or white, linear and judgmental.

Fortunately, as I sought out learning and growth, I began to grasp the concept of finding a gift in everything. This goes much deeper than natural preferences and normal times of disappointment and frustration. Being grateful means opening our minds and our hearts, non-judgmentally, to learning in every situation and always being thankful for what life brings. We become able to feel a feeling such as sadness and at the same time to be grateful for the richness of experience originating from a much deeper place than the impermanence of a feeling.

The importance of gratitude and living graciously, as we navigate our journey of healing from a diet and weight-obsessed life, is that nothing is left out. There are no exceptions such as "when I" or "if I". There is no back door or escape clause. With a grateful heart, there can be no denial, lack of acceptance, or failure.

C03

Instead, we experience natural consequences, feedback and learning — gifts in themselves.

If we lack gratitude and dwell in uncertainty and doubt, judgment and criticism, we may believe that wholeness and happiness will only happen when we reach a certain goal or when things on the outside change. If we wait to respect and love ourselves until some external goal is achieved, the message we send ourselves is that we are incomplete as we are and must be fixed, adjusted or changed somehow. When we live graciously, we honor all of life, living from trust strength, openness and an inner knowing that everything can be a vehicle for learning and all that is in our life is a gift.

Our purpose is to begin to welcome gratitude as a way of life and gracious living as the foundation of our journey. We explore being grateful for everything that happens — or doesn't happen — and learn to open our hearts and our lives to the beauty of life and the many gifts that are present.

CR

Gratitude and Gracious Living, Day 19

> *"Mimi, look! These thorns have a rose on the end!!"*
>
> —Lauren Smith, age 4

While similar words were stated quite eloquently in the 19th century by French poet Jean-Baptiste Alphonse Karr, *"Some people are always grumbling that roses have thorns. I am thankful that thorns have roses,"* my granddaughter, Lauren, had never heard the precious words of the poet when she uttered her discovery and delight. She was holding a rose to give to me, her grandmother ("Mimi"), and I realized at that moment how grateful I am for all that is in my life: my grandchildren, my grown children, such blessings — and this was before the accident in 2009 that nearly claimed my life.

My friends, I speak to you personally, now, with an open heart. I thought I knew gratitude until I was on life support, fighting for my life. Suddenly the touch of a cool wash cloth was heaven and the reassuring voice of my doctors, a gift greater than gold. I heard the voices of my children, grown up now but frightened; reaching into the depth of themselves for a maturity and a presence for which they were not prepared. They were by my side — strong and loving. I was never alone and I have never felt so wealthy.

What am I grateful for? Absolutely everything. I am healing now and I embrace each moment as a miracle and a gift. Yes, of course I know frustration, disappointment and sadness — and I also know the joy of a sunny morning, the taste of fresh berries, the warmth of my best friend's hug. I know it all because I am alive: grateful, beyond words.

Daily thoughts of gratitude can improve both your health and happiness by strengthening your immune system and increasing your level of optimism. Research shows that simply focusing each day on three to five things for which you can be grateful will increase your health and happiness. Everyone has something to be grateful for. Begin with two or three things you are grateful for and then build your gratitude list. Make your list and add to it each morning and each evening. Be sure to review your list often.

For an even stronger dose of health and happiness, express your gratitude to someone else. Holding the thought of gratitude for a good friend will benefit you. Expressing that gratitude to the friend will benefit both of you. Soon the "state" of gratitude will become a "trait" of gratefulness — a permanent personality aspect that benefits everyone.

MINDFULNESS ACTIVITY

If you started each day with gratitude, what three things would you list? If you ended each day with gratitude, what three things would you list? Is there something you might consider being grateful for that bothers you? Is there someone you might consider being grateful for who bothers you?

JOURNAL

Purposefully treat yourself with gratitude today: notice if your relationship with yourself changes. Each day for a week, begin and end your day with three "gratitudes". Are you able to look at a challenge as a gift? Please write about this.

ႠႥ

Gratitude and Gracious Living, Day 20

> *"Gratitude unlocks the fullness of life. It turns what we have into enough, and more. It turns denial into acceptance, chaos to order, confusion to clarity. It can turn a meal into a feast, a house into a home, a stranger into a friend. Gratitude makes sense of our past, brings peace for today, and creates a vision for tomorrow."*
>
> *—Melody Beattie*

Looking at your own life, what is precious? Can a gray day or some "bad news" be a source of delight or learning — in some way? You see, gratitude wants to be a verb — not a noun. Being grateful is a way of life, a path we choose. Yet how many of us think we'll be grateful when, well, we get what we want — or think we deserve? Is the very essence of life not enough? The holy life awaits and it is not about being religious. It is about walking the path before us with dignity, respect, learning, gratitude and love. It is about being a lifelong learner — living from the heart, being curious, unattached and open to outcome. Most of all, the holy life is right here, right now, offering itself to us each step of the way. We must listen deeply and speak our truth, trusting the next step and taking it with courage and love.

I am like you are: I want my life to be different, often. Looking out on the water where we live, I occasionally find myself longing to own one of the boats that float on Puget Sound — rather than being grateful for the beauty and the view. I do not need a boat to own. I know better. We all know better. And so I return to the moment and remind myself of all that is in my life and of the richness of this very moment and the next moment — and the next moment. You can too, I promise.

MINDFULNESS ACTIVITY

Have you believed at times that you will be happier when — or if? Is feeling grateful dependent upon something changing on the "outside"? What if you accepted yourself and your life as it is right now? Can you begin to find gratitude in the gift of an ordinary day? Are you able to name things of beauty surrounding you? Can you find an element of joy in a current sorrow?

JOURNAL

Please write about beauty in your life. Can you find beauty in the ordinary? What challenges can you name that contain the gift of joy? Are there times of "wanting" that might transform into gratitude with a small shift in perception?

CR

> *"Wisdom looks to see the jewel or flower shining beyond unexpected places or secured positions."*
>
> —*Spanish saying*

A significant shift occurs when we bring together the external world — that endless stream of stimulation provided by our physical, mental, emotional self — that we know well with the internal world — our unconscious or subconscious processes - we are not so sure of. The internal world is experienced in a way that does not lend itself to communication so our experience is often one of conflict.

How do we merge these two worlds and feel balanced and whole? They can seem so different and we often believe there is a barrier of some sort between our "inner life" and our "outer life". But what if an entire life awaits us by merging the two worlds? What if the true beauty of life exists by integrating our internal and external lives?

The poet Basho writes: *"Between our two lives, there is also the life of the cherry blossom."* Rather than either/or we are invited to experience our lives with grace and beauty as we learn to integrate what we call our "external" world with our "internal" world. Basho's "life of the cherry blossom" represents the exquisite and timeless essence of our true nature, which is found at the threshold between our two lives-the internal and external worlds. Until the two are integrated, the cherry blossom symbolizes the presence of a new world that we might touch, savor, and honor as we learn to expand our awareness and embrace all of who we are. We do this by resting in the ocean of our wholeness, knowing it is part of our journey to both want to reach for food to numb our feelings while at the same time to understand a choice based on wisdom is more appropriate in our journey toward eating and living mindfully.

Gratitude is our guide as we learn that our emotional eating is not our enemy but a rich message that reconnects us with the adventure and luscious experience of being alive. You see, it isn't the end result, the external gain or goal of thinness or control that will bring us happiness or tranquility. We experience happiness and tranquility as we are walking our path, as we are experiencing our lives moment by moment and making choices based on mindfulness and an aware presence. Trusting ourselves allows us to embrace difficulty, not eliminate it. And serenity and peace are available to us all along the way — no matter our doubt or uncertainty. As you take the next step on your path, may you breathe deeply, trusting the wisdom that speaks within you.

MINDFULNESS ACTIVITY

What do these words mean to you?

"Between our two lives, there is also the life of the cherry blossom."

Is there a conflict in your life that might be resolved by softening into a world that holds all possibility? Are you able to "define" who you are in the midst of "opposing forces"? Would you be willing to dedicate five minutes each day to do nothing but look at everything in your life as a gift?

CR

JOURNAL

Imagine the cherry blossom and write about it. Is there a hidden beauty in this struggle with eating or not eating? Are you able to sense the difference between either/or and a more expansive concept of both/and? In the meantime, can you touch and savor the life of the cherry blossom that holds our true nature? And how can gratitude enrich and nourish you as you explore and inquire? Will you commit to keeping gratitude a daily priority? Please write about your five-minute experience. Were you able to see the possibility of everything in life being a gift? Why or why not?

In Closing

Throughout this guidebook, you have experienced creative ideas for daily practical activities that invite mindful eating, resulting in increased health and wellness. Mindfulness, a foundation for a happy and fulfilling life, cultivates a sense of inner peace, understanding, trust and compassion. Some of the many benefits of a mindful life are increased acceptance, of self and others, and a life of freedom from the tyranny of critical thoughts and the resulting emotions. The ability to be aware of eating habits and to make healthful, life-affirming choices on a regular basis has been a rich beginning.

In a more expansive sense, each of us seeks peace, joy and freedom in the moments of our lives – whether food is involved or not. We long for the ability to open our eyes, our ears and our heart to a new and more fulfilling approach to our lives. Mindfulness is developing a clear mind and teaches us to look deeply at ourselves and at the world. Doing so, cultivating our ability to become mindfully aware, without judgment, can help reduce our response to stressful situations and improve the quality of our lives.

After experiencing *21 Days of Eating Mindfully*, you may have noticed how easy it is to spend most of your time either living in the past or thinking about the future. Though this is very common, the behavior of reflecting on past memories or fantasizing about future events robs us of our one true experience in life: the gift of the present moment. Mindfulness is the awareness that emerges through paying attention on purpose, in the present moment, non-judgmentally to life just as it is. Mindfulness means paying attention to things as they actually are

CR

in any given moment and to do so with fierce compassion and a loving heart.

So, with mindfulness as our companion and our guide, let's take a look at HEALING – at the seven components of *21 Days of Eating Mindfully* and imagine how each "letter" could be a lesson, not only in eating mindfully, but in living a mindful life.

HUNGER AND HEALING

What do you hunger for in your life? Ask yourself: what do I want? What is my vision for my life? What steps are involved in realizing this vision? Then take the first step. Regardless of our nationality, language or personal taste, just as we need food so do we need emotional nourishment: love, kindness, appreciation and acceptance from others and from ourselves. We need to find our place in the world. And we need to address and satisfy our need for happiness, peace of mind and freedom.

Our relationship to food can be our teacher, informing us about who we are, what we value and how we might live, give and love from our deepest level of being. Can you expand your awareness to involve more than what is on your plate or what isn't and allow feelings and thoughts to emerge that had previously been avoided in some way? What can you learn? What life lessons might be near? Can you gently accept this new information with loving acceptance of yourself?

EMPATHY AND EMOTIONAL EATING

Stop for a moment and ask yourself: have I been resisting painful feelings or thoughts – perhaps for a long time in my life? If so, your efforts are only natural and are simply a heroic attempt at feeling "better" or feeling good about yourself. What we long for, I believe, is the ability to be fully present with ourselves, no matter what. Again, this skill is called mindfulness and it asks us to accept ourselves, with understanding and compassion, from moment to moment.

If how we eat is how we live, what might we learn about ourselves? And if our core beliefs about being alive are reflected in our eating habits, what might these core beliefs be? Can you tease apart the eating behaviors from the beliefs and values that are foundational to how you act and behave? Often when we eat emotionally, something deeper is asking for our attention. With a compassionate and non-judgmental heart, it is possible to allow our present habits to illuminate the areas in ourselves in need of healing.

When we are able to pause an automatic behavior – even for a moment – we are opening a door to healing. When we open this door, we have the opportunity to make a choice rather than rely on automatic and engrained behavior. Would you be willing to make an agreement with yourself to stop before you reach for food and, instead of eating something mindlessly, simply feel your feelings? Can you trust yourself enough to welcome what presents itself? Developing the practice of pausing, in itself, invites mindful awareness. And it is with awareness, presence, that health in body, mind and spirit are possible.

AWARENESS AND ACCEPTANCE

Mindfulness asks of us to bring a loving acceptance to who we are and to our lives, just as they are right now. Rather than continue a life of mindlessness or automatic pilot, we learn to bring a mindful awareness to our days, our moments and our choices. All healing

☙

begins with awareness. There is a person within who wants authentic expression, love and acceptance.

With few exceptions, in childhood we are not taught to be okay with ourselves – to love and accept ourselves as we are. Most of us have brought a belief into our adult years that we must do something to be "better". We believe we must fix ourselves, strive and achieve rather than meet the person inside and love who we find. It is possible, though, to open our hearts once again and through forgiveness and mercy, begin to heal.

Can you quiet your mind for a few moments and listen to your body? Can you become aware and curious, cultivating a state of mindfulness and tender self-acceptance? It is awareness and acceptance, graciousness toward ourselves, that changes perspective and invites us to respond to life with an open and non-judgmental heart. When we honor ourselves in this way, we begin to fully embrace our feelings, our experiences and our lives.

LOVING AND LETTING BE

In getting to know the part of us that, at times, overeats or eats poorly, we have an opportunity to look beneath the voices that tell us we are guilty and unacceptable. Here, we find the person who is trying, as best, to avoid distressing thoughts or feelings. We have a chance to get to know and accept this person. We have an opportunity to create a healing relationship with this person who has only done her best, all along. And the way of this healing relationship is love.

Love is accepting, honoring and forgiving. It is patient and deeply understanding. It is love that sees what is and does not demand change, asking only for acceptance of who we are and for what is happening at the time...without judgment. As the poet Mark Nepo says: "Loving yourself requires us to believe in and stay loyal to something no one else can see...our own self-worth."

Again, ask yourself: does my life reflect my deepest values? Am I able to say with full agreement, "Yes, I love well"? Am I willing to love myself, right now, just the way I am? And if not, what will it take? Is there a tendency to want to move away from certain thoughts? Can all thoughts be welcomed as visitors, and then let them move on?

Letting go of former ideas and strongly held beliefs about ourselves– ones that are neither healthful nor honoring to who we are – is a part of loving ourselves. Cultivating a "letting go" or a "letting be" is essential to practicing mindful living. First we allow our thoughts to be present. We simply observe them, impartially. And then, we simply let thoughts float on by, like clouds in the sky. Perhaps we may notice impermanence – how each thought changes. In time, loving and letting be can become a way of life, a way of living our lives in acceptance and with full presence.

INQUIRY AND INTENTION

In healing, it becomes necessary to delve, discover and end our dysfunctional ideas about ourselves and our outdated ways of behaving in our lives. This must be done with great love and tenderness. First we must accept what we find – as we search within – and then allow our findings to be something we learn from rather than one more thing to be criticized.

Our purpose is to cultivate curiosity about our lives and about ourselves. The quality of our inquiry will determine the depth of

CR

our healing. As we define and commit to what we want for ourselves, our lives begin to open up...to become more majestic and beautiful. We are able to live by intention and in full engagement with our lives, no matter what our circumstances or history.

All change begins with where we are right now. Mindfulness is paying attention on purpose. It is creating awareness without judgment or criticism. All inquiry begins with mindful self-knowledge and self-acceptance. Intention is what we do next: how we choose to live based on our discoveries. Ask yourself one more time:

Am I showing up fully in my life – holding nothing back?

Am I paying attention to what has heart and meaning to me – letting the rest "be"?

Am I open to outcome – trusting emergence – or I am in reaction to what emerges?

Am I telling my own truth, without blame or judgment – or am I holding others responsible?

What do you truly want for your life? You must be willing to take the risk to explore deeply, allowing your comfort zone to be a memory. Ask yourself: "What do I want more than anything in my life?" and then listen to the whispers of your heart. Start with an overall truth, such as 'I want to be kinder' and then break it down, step by step. Kinder than what? Where am I now and where do I go next in being a kinder person? Or try it backwards: start with a small step and see where it leads...how it is related to a grander vision for your life. For example, set an intention to walk 15

CR

minutes a day and discover the role activity plays in your vision for wellness and well-being.

NURTURE AND NOURISHMENT

We have talked about healthy nourishment and though it is important to wellness and well-being, reaching the heart of the matter is what will bring healing. Learning to nurture ourselves is the key to learning how to truly nourish our bodies, our minds and spirits. And it is a nourished person who will discover wholeness and joy.

There can be no effective personal nurture, no true wellness, without first accepting and honoring who we are and why we behave the way we do. We are not broken and we are not to blame for our actions. We have tried, heroically, to cover wounds and prevent unwelcomed feelings and experiences. Perhaps it is time to find our way back to ourselves and to what we truly need. My belief is we need to be all that we are and to live an authentic and wholehearted life. That means we learn to trust ourselves and do nothing but what is in our own best interest. It means we feel our feelings and welcome our thoughts - accepting all that is here in the present moment.

Nurturing and nourishing ourselves means we find ways of caring for ourselves that do not involve eating inappropriately. Our bodies depend upon nutritional nourishment; our souls depend upon nurture and self-care. The need for nurturance is a human need. With acceptance and honoring of ourselves, we learn and grow. With forgiveness and a kind heart, we let love heal – as many times a day as it takes. With compassion, we find our way back to ourselves.

CR

GRATITUDE AND GRACIOUS LIVING

Can you feel it? Gratitude? If not, can you imagine being grateful for everything, regardless? The importance of gratitude and of living a gracious life is that there is no back door clause. There are no exceptions such as "when I lose weight" or "when I finish my tasks". And this is a gift. If we allow ourselves a way out, we will probably find it. If we realize that all we need is right here, right now...in some way...there can be no denial, lack of acceptance, or failure. We begin to live a life of meaning and joy.

Research shows that simply focusing on three to five things each day that bring you happiness will increase your health and well-being. To increase the impact of gratitude, express what you are grateful for to someone else. Make their day! Soon this "state" of gratitude will become a "trait" and you will find yourself feeling grateful naturally. At the same time, the immune system strengthens and you will be less likely to experience long lasting depression or a relapse of depression.

Looking at your own life, what is precious to you? Can some bit of "bad" news or a disappointment be a source of learning or appreciation in some way? Can you imagine welcoming everything in life? Once again, I speak to you from my heart. I thought I was grateful until I was unable to move in the ICU unit in a large trauma center, having been run over by an SUV. I was fighting for my life. I remember the sound of my daughter's voice, calm and reassuring, loving and mature. As she placed a cool cloth on my forehead, I felt such relief. My sons, grown up now, were by my side - the sound of their voices like music. And if this weren't enough, my three grandchildren, my husband and beautiful daughter-in-law, all there, loving, caring and praying. I was alive and I was going to recover. Gratitude.

CR

And now, two years later, when I am stuck in traffic or bored on the treadmill, I remember to find the gift...to be grateful. Do I still get caught up in less-than-gracious living? Of course. The difference is that I know what to do now and how to shift my thinking. I don't have to like everything to be grateful and neither do you. Gratitude simply asks us to consider ...to open to the possibility of ...our lives being deeply blessed, no matter our circumstances, and that our hearts can always make room for gracious living.

With all of the self inquiry, mindfulness activities and journaling you have done, you will have learned many things about yourself — perhaps some things you weren't aware of until now. Is what you envision for yourself different from the 'story' you tell yourself? What if you changed the old story and scripted a new one, fresh and current, loving and compassionate?

Here is my suggestion for capturing all you have learned so far: in addition to your journal (which you will hopefully continue writing in), create a "vision board", a simple yet powerful visualization tool. Start with a corkboard or a large piece of strong paper to display pictures, symbols and/or representations of your vision for your life on. Feel free to dream BIG! Open the door to the world and its abundance and let your wishes begin.

Start by making a list, jotting down what you want in your life. Then start gathering meaningful pictures and inspiring words and phrases that resonate with your vision (from favorite magazines, the Internet, etc.) and begin to cut and paste. When selecting your materials, consider areas of your life including health and wellness, fitness, wealth, nourishment, hobbies, family, relationships, etc. Feel free to create — this is your vision for your life. Treat it with honor and joy. And above all, have fun with the experience!

When your vision board is complete, reread your journal entries. Pause and allow the lessons to sink in once again, and open to what you have learned about yourself in these 21 days. Trusting yourself, listen deeply to what your inner voice has to say and let truth speak.

Step back from your vision board and gaze at your creation. What do you see? Do you want to add anything — or eliminate something? What lessons are evident for you?

Now, with compassion and a loving heart, allow a weaving of the lessons to emerge. Begin to create your own personal eating guidelines — living guidelines — from your newly expanded awareness, acceptance, inquiry, health, nourishment, love and gratitude. Let your guidelines serve you on your journey to becoming all that you are and living your life with boldness, strength, clarity, passion and deep love.[84]

In closing, I would like to quote my own teacher of mindfulness, Dr. Jon Kabat-Zinn, who states in his book Mindfulness for Beginners: reclaiming the present moment and your life: *"Mindfulness as a practice provides endless opportunities to cultivate greater intimacy with your own mind and to tap into and develop your deep interior resources for learning, growing, healing, and potentially for transforming your understanding of who you are and how you might live more wisely and with greater well-being, meaning, and happiness in this world."*

CR

Recommended Reading

My commitment is to work from my heart and to honor the sacredness of your process. To that end, I have hand-selected the following resources to support you on your journey. For additional recommended reading, or to purchase any of these books, please visit the "Eating Mindfully" book list on the Resources page of the Simple Serenity website, www.simpleserenity.com.

The Yoga of Eating: Transcending Diets and Dogma to Nourish the Natural Self
by Charles Eisenstein

Intuitive Eating: A Revolutionary Program That Works
by Evelyn Tribole and Elise Resch

Women, Food and God: An Unexpected Path to Almost Everything
by Geneen Roth

When Food Is Food and Love Is Love: A Step-by-Step Spiritual Program to Break Free from Emotional Eating
by Geneen Roth

Breaking Free from Emotional Eating
by Geneen Roth

The Fourfold Way: Walking the Paths of the Warrior, Teacher, Healer, and Visionary
by Angeles Arrien

Meditations from the Mat: Daily Reflections on the Path of Yoga

by Rolf Gates and Katrina Kenison

The Book of Awakening: Having the Life You Want by Being Present to the Life You Have

by Mark Nepo

The Happiness Project: Or, Why I Spent a Year Trying to Sing in the Morning, Clean My Closets, Fight Right, Read Aristotle, and Generally Have More Fun

by Gretchen Rubin

Full Catastrophe Living: Using the Wisdom of Your Body and Mind to Face Stress, Pain, and Illness

by Jon Kabat-Zinn

Wherever You Go There You Are

by Jon Kabat-Zinn

ଔ

Appendix A

> *"Tell me what you eat, and I will tell you what you are."*
>
> *—Jean Anthelme Brillat-Savarin (1755-1826)*

To enrich your journey, the following URL provides you with exclusive access to 21 days of videos, audio files and PDFs: simpleserenity.com/eating-mindfully/21-days.php

H: Hunger and Healing Overview (video)

Day 1 Guidelines for eating mindfully | eating mindfully means no more dieting (audio)

Day 2 Mindful eating exercise

Day 3 Mindful transitions

E: Empathy and Emotional Eating Overview (video)

Day 4 Food for thought

Day 5 Mindful meal practices

Day 6 Guide to responding rather than reacting to emotion

A: Awareness and Acceptance Overview (video)

Day 7 Five-minute mindfulness meditation (audio)

Day 8 Ten Ways to Love Yourself

Day 9 Six steps to overcoming a challenge

℞

L: Love and Letting Be Overview (video)

Day 10 Why diets don't work

Day 11 Loving kindness meditation (audio)

Day 12 Awareness meditation (audio)

I: Inquiry and Intention Overview (video)

Day 13 Setting a healing intention

Day 14 A prayer for kindness

Day 15 Guided imagery for relaxation (audio)

N: Nurture and Nourishment Overview (video)

Day 16 Healthy nourishment

Day 17 Changing your story: over-indulgence | deprivation (audio)

Day 18 Becoming an optimist

G: Gratitude and Gracious Living Overview (video)

Day 19 Gratitude = better health

Day 20 "Here we go" (audio)

Day 21 Recipe for gratitude

ℭ

Appendix B

1 My commitment is to work from my heart and to honor the sacredness of your process. To support you on your journey, *21 Days of Eating Mindfully* includes 21 days of bonus handouts, videos and audio files that can be accessed daily at: simpleserenity.com/eating-mindfully/21-days.php
I also encourage you to explore other books, articles and DVDs on the subject and have hand-selected the following resources: simpleserenity.com/resources.php

2 Learn more about the power of a vision board here: livingmindfullytoday.com/2011/02/03/mindful-practices/creating-a-vision-board/

3 Dietary Guidelines for Americans is available free at: health.gov/dietaryguidelines/dga2010/DietaryGuidelines2010.pdf
For more information, tips and tools, visit: choosemyplate.gov/

4 Learn more about the power of a vision board here: livingmindfullytoday.com/2011/02/03/mindful-practices/creating-a-vision-board/

simpleserenity.com | livingmindfullytoday.com

Made in the USA
Charleston, SC
18 November 2012